I0467668

Introduction

Mesothelioma is a type of cancer which is associated with high and prolonged sin the mesothelium (the protective membrane that surrounds most of the body's internal organs).

The cancer is commonly found in the outer lining of the lungs (pleura), the inside lining of the abdominal cavity (peritoneum), and the sac that surrounds the heart (pericardium). The two most common types of mesothelioma are pleural and peritoneal.

Who is at Risk?

Exposure to asbestos is a significant risk factor. People who have worked in jobs where they have been exposed asbestos and family members of these workers who have had second-hand exposure are both at risk for the development of mesothelioma.

Although still considered as a rare type of cancer, about 2,000 new cases of mesothelioma are diagnosed in the US annually. Men outnumbered women, but both can develop the disease, regardless of age. About 70 to 80 percent of the patients have a history of prolonged exposure to asbestos particles at work. However, not all cases are related to asbestos.

Exposure to Asbestos

Asbestos is a natural mineral composed of durable and fire-resistant fibers used commercially in industries including shipbuilding, textiles, insulation, heating and construction, roofing and flooring, automotive repair, and much more. Asbestos was used as ceiling tiles in old school buildings. Since the late 1800s, asbestos was mined continuously and widely used on Navy ships. It was only in the 1970s that the government started regulating the use of asbestos.

Mesothelioma Symptoms and Options for Treatment

Symptoms of mesothelioma typically appear until 30 to 50 years after exposure to asbestos occurred. They often resemble signs of other ailments, so mesothelioma is often difficult to diagnose without knowing the history of the patient and several medical tests (such as CT scan, x-ray, biopsy, MRI, and so on). Common symptoms may include: chest pain, weight loss, fever, shortness of breath, swelling, and pain. Standard treatment options include: chemotherapy, radiation, and surgery

Thanks for downloading this book, It is my sincere believe it will answer all your questions.

Table of Contents

Mesothelioma: The Silent Killer

It has been known for years that asbestos is harmful to humans and mesothelioma is preventable. Despite this knowledge, thousands of Americans have suffered from the damaging effects of asbestos exposure. Before getting into the details of mesothelioma, it is critical for you to know that if you or someone you love has mesothelioma or has died from it, a mesothelioma attorney should be contacted immediately.

There is a good chance that a mesothelioma lawyer will be able to help you determine whether the death or illness meets the stipulations to be filed as a mesothelioma lawsuit and whether you may be entitled to a mesothelioma settlement. This agreement can go a long way in helping a family pay for treatments for the disease as well as funeral costs, in the event of death.

A mesothelioma diagnosis is made when a cancerous tumor has invaded the mesothelium cells of an organ. This type of tumor is most commonly found in lungs, heart and abdominal cells and is caused by direct exposure to asbestos and asbestos related products. The most predominant form of mesothelioma is pleural mesothelioma, which is an extraordinarily rare, vicious kind of lung cancer. There are two classes of pleural mesothelioma - diffuse and malignant (cancerous) and benign (not cancerous).

Statistics indicate that malignant mesothelioma is a severe form of the disease and accounts for about 75% of all instances of mesothelioma. Malignant mesothelioma is so aggressive it requires fair treatment not only because of the type of cancer it is but, a forceful response to treatment is needed because, by the time this form of mesothelioma is diagnosed, the disease has progressed into an advanced form of cancer. Mesothelioma diagnosis is made through biopsy and a pathological study.

As the tumor spreads over the pleura of the lung, it causes the lung's outer lining to thicken and lose elasticity. The growth of the tumor creates a progressively restraining type of rubber band around the lung, and as the lung becomes more constricted; it begins to become smaller resulting in an inability to perform its functions.

A standard initial indicator or sign that someone has mesothelioma is when they exhibit shortness of breath following being involved in exercise such as doing yard work, walking, lifting, etc. As mesothelioma advances, with the lung(s) becoming less efficient due to the tumors, the patient will begin to evidence shortness of breath during activities requiring little exertion. In time, the shortness of breath will occur during periods of lying down, sitting and resting.

As the growth of the tumor starts to move inward, the lung becomes even more constricted. As the growth begins to move to nearby tissue such as in the chest cavity and around the ribs, the level of pain patients experience can be excruciating.

There is not good news about malignant mesothelioma because, at this point in time, there is not a cure. The prognosis is directly related to the size of the tumor, the stage of growth, the specific form of cell the tumor is comprised of and the tumor's response to interventions and treatments.

Another form of mesothelioma is peritoneal mesothelioma, which attacks the peritoneum membrane of several abdominal organs. Peritoneum mesothelioma is charged with being accountable for almost 20% of the cases of mesothelioma/year. Although peritoneal mesothelioma is not as rare as pleural mesothelioma, it presents more aggressively and results in a shortened life expectancy. Peritoneal mesothelioma can be benign or malignant. Because this type of cancer takes years to develop, it very often is found by sheer chance and prior to symptoms beginning to be apparent.

Symptoms of peritoneal mesothelioma include abdominal pain, generalized weakness, loss of appetite and subsequent loss of weight, nausea, and swelling of the abdomen. The symptoms of peritoneal mesothelioma progress slowly and as time passes become more severe. Like pleural mesothelioma, there is no cure and the prognosis is affected by such things as the tumor size and stage of development, the cell type of the tumor, and the tumor's response to treatment.

What Are The Symptoms Of Mesothelioma Cancer?

If you would like to know what the symptoms of mesothelioma cancer are, the following information might just be what you were looking for. First, if somebody is trying to find out the more about this incredibly deadly form of cancer, more than likely either they are concerned that they might have it, or someone they know may have contracted it.

If that is the case, you should stop doing research on the internet immediately. What you need to be doing instead is to schedule an appointment with your doctor, and arrange for medical tests to be done that can either confirm or deny your suspicions.

One of the main reasons that mesothelioma cancer is so lethal is that it usually is not diagnosed in its very early stages. All cancers are graded according to their development. These are called stage I, stage II, or stage III.

Most mesothelioma cancer patients only discover that they have it when it gets to stage III. Unfortunately, by this time in most cases it is too late for the doctors to effectively treat you.

A few of the reasons for this is that your body is no longer healthy enough to take some of the grueling treatments used on people with this disease, it has spread throughout your body and nothing at all can be done, or the tumor is so large, that an operation is impossible.

It is highly recommended that if you think you are experiencing mesothelioma cancer symptoms that you let your physician know of your fears. Otherwise, you might be treated for a disease or illness, which has identical symptoms. Most family doctors will never have had a patient that had this form of cancer in their entire professional career. In other words, they are not familiar with it, and usually do not diagnose it correctly on your initial visit to their office.

The following are a few of the most common symptoms of mesothelioma cancer, persistent cough, shortness of breath, or chest pain. By reading those symptoms, it is very easy even for the layperson to see, that these are the same complaints that a person can and does make for all kinds of other ordinary ailments, like pneumonia. Some of the less common symptoms are a high fever that does not go away, extreme weight loss, or sweating a great deal while you are sleeping at night.

Thankfully, just because you have any or all of the above symptoms, does not mean that you have mesothelioma cancer. But, as the old saying goes, "It is better to be safe than sorry", and when it comes to this form of cancer, there has never been a better expression to heed.

Everything You Should Know About Mesothelioma Treatment Options

The continuous exposure to asbestos results in the cancerous condition called Mesothelioma. If you do not treat this disease in time, then it might prove to be deadly. You need to take corrective treatment of Mesothelioma. If you have been exposed to asbestos, you should choose an extensive medical check-up. The situations of Mesothelioma have been enhanced on a daily basis. You will locate Mesothelioma treatment choices. You need to go for the best one. From this post, you will certainly learn every little thing about Mesothelioma therapy options.

Before you go with Mesothelioma therapy, the first thing that you have to do is find out whether you are dealing with Mesothelioma or not. The symptoms of Mesothelioma are chest discomfort, stomach pain, coughing, fat burning, body ache, etc. If you have any of these indicators, you need to start the Mesothelioma treatment.

Chemotherapy, medication, and radiations are the most preferred types of Mesothelioma therapies. The Mesothelioma treatment options will differ from one person to yet another. Those who are in the early stages can easily opt for easy medication. However, if you have been detected with this condition since very long time back, you have to complete treatment of Mesothelioma.

The Mesothelioma therapy choices will certainly be of fantastic help to the Mesothelioma victims. The nature of the treatment of Mesothelioma will identify the cost of the Mesothelioma treatment. The treatment will get costly if the patient is in the final stage of the disease. But if you have merely been detected with Mesothelioma, it will not be that expensive.

The details on Mesothelioma therapy choices can be gotten from a multitude of sources. An excellent internet site can be gone to by you to get the Mesothelioma info. It is your obligation to try to find a great and trustworthy website. It is extremely necessary to choose Mesothelioma therapy. The Mesothelioma treatment has conserved multitude of Mesothelioma patients. You will locate good info on Mesothelioma treatment options from the net.

Any person who has managed asbestos in their lives should acquire Mesothelioma treatment information even if the illness is not pinpointed. This is due to the reality that the illness can easily not be recognized for many years, even if a person gets infected and it takes time for the illness to come to be serious. Mesothelioma treatment info can be acquired from many sources like books, magazines, specialists and the net. It will be rather valuable if one gets the details from as numerous sources as possible. In that manner, you will certainly understand, should in case you are pinpointed with the illness.

You can easily first read some books and magazines. You can search the internet next. You will come across some

Mesothelioma therapy info posted by experts on the subject. You can inspect those out very carefully. When you get some idea, you may then ask your doctor about Mesothelioma therapy details.

The stages of Mesothelioma are divided into four categories. If the illness is detected in the early stages, then there is a far better opportunity for a quick recovery. The three kinds of typical treatment, procedure are surgical treatment, chemotherapy, and radiation. The manner of therapy depends on the stages of the illness. And the decision will certainly be made by the physician after taking a look at the client's documents. In this instance, it is you.

At present, researchers and doctors are doing medical examinations on customers. However, only selected patients may go through these examinations. This is since the experiments are not totally a success yet. So, the consent of customer and family members is needed. The experiments are done on the customers only after the needed paperwork is finished These brand-new tests are part of chemotherapy medicine, and there seems some success. If it becomes fully successful, then it would mean a great deal to both Mesothelioma patients and researchers.

Mesothelioma therapy info ought to be discovered by everybody who has been in close link with asbestos now or before. This will make an individual continue to be calm both mentally and emotionally.

Mesothelioma Staging Systems-How Do You Stage Mesothelioma

Most known cancers have various staging systems which have been developed to aid doctors and physicians in the diagnosis and treatment of individual cases of cancer.

Pleural mesothelioma is the only form of mesothelioma that has been successfully staged as it is the commonest type of the disease. There are three different staging systems used to determine the extent of pleural mesothelioma, each one of these three different staging system measures different aspects of cancer, including the size of the tumor, the level of spreading {metastases} and the probable involvement of lymph nodes.

The stage of mesothelioma at the time of diagnosis determines to an enormous extent the type of treatment prescribed by the doctor.

Butchart System

The Butchart System is the oldest staging system for malignant mesothelioma and is the one most commonly used by doctors and specialists to diagnose and treat the tumor. The Butchart System is based on the tumor size (mass) and divides malignant mesothelioma into four stages:

* Stage 1 - Malignant mesothelioma has affected the right or left side of the chest cavity (pleural lining) and may be seen in the diaphragm.

* Stage 2 - Malignant mesothelioma has been found in the pleura on both sides of the body and may have also moved into the heart, stomach, or esophagus on both sides. Lymph nodes may be affected.

* Stage 3 - Malignant mesothelioma has reached the abdominal cavity (peritoneum). Lymph nodes past the chest may be affected.

* Stage 4 - Malignant mesothelioma has reached other organs and has entered the blood stream.

TNM System

The TNM System is a more modern staging system for malignant mesothelioma. The TNM System is based on the extent of the tumor, metastasis, and lymph node involvement. Again, the TNM System divides malignant mesothelioma into four stages:

* Stage 1 - Malignant mesothelioma is present in the left or right chest cavity (pleura) and may have metastasized to the lung, the

sac around the heart (pericardium) or the diaphragm on the same side. Lymph nodes in stage 1 are not involved.

* Stage 2 - Malignant mesothelioma has reached from one side of the chest cavity to a lymph node near the lung area on the same side as cancer. Cancer has metastasized to the diaphragm, pericardium (sac around the heart), or the lung on the same side as the primary tumor.

* Stage 3 - Malignant mesothelioma has penetrated the chest lining, heart, esophagus, muscle, ribs and vital organs within the chest cavity on the same side as cancer. Lymph nodes may or may not be involved during this stage.

* Stage 4 - Malignant mesothelioma has metastasized to the pleural area and the lymph nodes on the opposite side of where the cancerous tumor is located. It may also have reached the chest cavities or lungs on both sides, or may have spread to the abdomen.

Brigham System

The Brigham System is the most modern of the three malignant mesothelioma staging systems. The Brigham System looks at different variables such as the involvement of the lymph nodes and the surgical ability to remove a malignant mesothelioma tumor (resectability). For this reason, it is not used very often to stage mesothelioma, as the cancer is rarely operable. The Brigham System divides malignant mesothelioma into four stages:

* Stage 1 - Malignant mesothelioma tumor is still resectable (able to be removed surgically), and the lymph nodes are not affected.

* Stage 2 - Malignant mesothelioma tumor is still resectable, but the lymph nodes are now affected.

* Stage 3 - Malignant mesothelioma tumor is not resectable, and the malignant mesothelioma has penetrated the heart, chest wall, abdominal cavity or diaphragm. Lymph nodes may or may not be affected.

* Stage 4 - Malignant mesothelioma tumor is not resectable and has completely metastasized (spread throughout the body).

Process of Staging Malignant Mesothelioma

When mesothelioma is diagnosed by a physician or specialist, they must determine the extent of cancer and how far it has spread. Most often, they will use imaging procedures to see inside the chest or abdomen to help determine the stage of the malignant mesothelioma. The imaging options physicians may use include:

* Chest X-ray

* CT scan of the chest and abdomen

* MRI scan of the chest and abdomen

* PET of the chest and abdomen.

A Brief Overview of Alternative Treatments for Prostate Cancer

While prostate cancer is often treated with surgery, radiation or hormone therapy, alternative treatments for prostate cancer should be considered before undergoing these potentially dangerous treatments. Since prostate cancer cells grow at a very slow rate, it is possible to treat this cancer by adjusting your lifestyle and diet.

The orthodox treatments of prostate cancer include radiotherapy, androgen deprivation therapy, and prostatectomy. Each of these treatments carries a significant risk. Radiotherapy is the use of radiation to treat the prostate cancer. Androgen deprivation therapy involves either castration or estrogen hormone replacement therapy. Lastly, a prostatectomy is the removal of the prostate gland itself. Radiotherapy involves the use of radiation to treat cancer, which always carries the risk of contracting radiation poison or even another form of cancer.

Androgen deprivation, whether by castration or estrogen replacement therapy, will reduce the male sex drive and cause impotence in the case of castration. A prostatectomy, among other side effects, has been shown to cause impotence in 60% of patients, and incontinence in 39% of patients. It is for these reasons, then, that an alternative treatment for prostate cancer should be considered if you are diagnosed with prostate cancer.

Prostate cancer is particular in that its cancer cells grow at a very slow rate. What this means is that alternative treatments for prostate cancer are not only viable but could be preferable. So what are these alternative treatments? The most significant factors are your lifestyle and diet. Some studies have shown that diet alone has caused prostate cancer in patients, due to unhealthy food selection. Eating the right foods in itself can be thought of as an alternative treatment for prostate cancer. It is important to know which foods to avoid, as well as what you should be eating.

Pig meat that isn't fully cooked or that has been saved and refrigerated may contain a fungus that produces a toxin shown to cause different kinds of cancers. Cooking the meat will kill this fungus. Thus, one should never eat, for example, cold bacon or sausage. Peanuts, cashews, barley, mushrooms and even corn can contain certain carcinogenic fungi as well.

Regardless of all the alternative treatments for prostate cancer, the food you ingest is either going to have a positive or negative effect on your chosen alternative treatment. Foods that will have a positive effect include mostly fruits and vegetables: raspberries, strawberries, broccoli, carrots, almonds, pineapple and similar foods. Whenever possible, it is best to avoid cooking the fruits and vegetables, as this kills their cancer-fighting enzymes and reduces their effectiveness at treating any cancer.

Watchful waiting may also be called expectant management, observation, and active surveillance. What exactly does watchful waiting mean? Well, what it doesn't mean is to ignore the warning signs of a high PSA. What it does mean is working with your doctor to set up a protocol that includes regular monitoring of your PSA.

Some doctors may prefer to closely monitor your prostate, and some may describe a less intensive approach. Using a variety of methods such as the PSA blood test, digital rectal exams, biopsies, and ultrasounds, it's possible to carefully monitor your cancer and take action if there is a change in your test results.

I should point out here that like most men my prostate and the idea of being constantly examined didn't appeal to me. After all, we're talking about a most intimate part of the male anatomy. This being the case, it's critical to find a doctor who you feel comfortable with and who is willing to answer your questions and discuss all the options.

With active surveillance or watchful waiting, only men whose cancer is growing will be treated. For men with lower PSA, this means avoiding the many side effects of aggressive procedures such as surgery. Of course, if you go the route of watchful waiting there is the danger that the cancer will spread. If this happens then, your treatment options may become limited.

Older men, especially those with other serious health problems watchful is a viable alternative. But for younger men who are in good health and who have many years ahead of them a more aggressive treatment plan is probably the best choice.

Whichever option you choose watchful waiting, or more aggressive intervention remember these points. First of all, unless your cancer, when detected, is in an advanced stage, you have time to carefully consider your opinions. Secondly, find a doctor you are comfortable with and that you trust. Thirdly weigh all the options and if watchful waiting is for you follow your doctor's advice and make sure you monitor your PSA on a regular schedule.

Information-Your Number Key For Coping With Mesothelioma Cancer

After you receive a diagnosis of mesothelioma, you number one priority should be to get adequate information about the disease so that you can make the right informed decisions on the necessary steps you need to take.

When looking for information about mesothelioma cancer, first know what type of mesothelioma you have,the pleural mesothelioma is the commonest, but there are also other types of mesothelioma depending on the part of the body that is affected by the cancer. Talk with your health care team. Ask them for information about your specific type of cancer, including the cell type and the stage (extent) of your cancer. This is helpful because your cancer treatment will be designed just for you.

The stage of the cancer, as well as other factors, will help determine the goal of treatment. Most types of mesothelioma cancer treatment have some goals; provide a cure, control the disease, or ease symptoms of the cancer and help make the patient comfortable. Sometimes the treatment goal changes after the treatment starts. Talk with your doctor, and make sure you understand what your treatment options are, so you can make the best decisions for you and your family.

We live in an information-packed age. Cancer information can be complex and confusing. To find accurate and up-to-date information, use reliable sources, such as journals or Web sites from well-respected cancer centers, national cancer organizations, health professional organizations.One good source of information is www.mesotheliomacorner.blogspot.com; you will find the necessary information you need in a very easy to understand manner.

Look for information that has been reviewed by medical experts, is updated often, and states the purpose of the information. When you get information, discuss it with your healthcare team to find out if and how it applies to you. Remember, written information cannot take the place of medical advice from your doctor or cancer care team.

Getting information from your health care team

Learning all they can about you and your cancer is the first step your health care team will take. A biopsy and other lab tests, physical exams, and imaging tests will be done to figure out the stage (extent) of your cancer. Next, your doctor uses all of this information to narrow down options and recommend treatment. Your doctor may talk with other doctors and health care professionals to help plan your treatment. You may also wish to get a second opinion at another treatment center. Getting a second opinion may help you feel more comfortable when deciding on your best treatment option.

Talking to doctors, nurses, and other members of the health care team is very important for people diagnosed with cancer. Your health care team can tell you where to look for information about your type of cancer and its treatment. They can answer your questions, give you support, and refer you to community resources. Allow yourself to take in information at your own pace. You decide when you are ready to talk when you want to learn more about your cancer, and how much you want to learn.

Ask questions

Doctors and nurses are good sources of information when you have medical questions. Before appointments, write down any questions you may have about your type of cancer, treatment, side effects, and any limits on the activity you might have during treatment. Other members of your health care team, such as pharmacists, dietitians, social workers, physical therapists, and radiation therapists are experts in different areas. Don't be afraid to ask them questions, too. Asking questions show you want to learn and take an active role in your treatment. If the health care team member does not have time to answer all of your questions, ask when a good time would be to finish your conversation or ask about other ways to get the answers you need.

Know how to reach your doctor at any time

People with cancer must know when they need to call the doctor. Ask which side effects or unusual signs need to be reported right away. Some things can wait until the next office visit, or until regular office hours when you can call and speak to a nurse. But if you have severe or unexpected side effects, you need to know how to reach your doctor when the office is closed. Be sure you have this phone number and that your loved ones have it, too.

Family members may wish to speak with members of your health care team. This can help them answer questions and find support to deal with their feelings. Your health care team is bound by law to keep information about your health confidential. They will not discuss your health status with family members and friends, unless you give your written permission for them to do so. Let your doctors and nurses know which family members and friends may be contacting them and with whom they can share information.

Feel at ease with your health care team

Ideally, a health caregiver should be patient, understanding, have all the time in the world to answer questions, and know how to explain things to you so you could easily understand, finding all of this in most health professionals is rare. Most times if you find most of the qualities you want in your health team you will just have to cope with the other little missing deficiencies.Still, it is important for you to trust your doctor and other members of the health care team. If you feel a lack of trust and open communication is keeping you from getting good medical care, ask for a referral to another doctor with whom you feel more comfortable. Also, don't be afraid to ask your doctor for a referral for a second opinion. You will need to be an active member of your healthcare team. As an active team member, you will need to do things like keeping your scheduled appointments, take medicines as prescribed, and report side effects.

Treating Mesothelioma after Surgery, Chemotherapy or Radiation

Asbestos is a toxic fibrous mineral that is naturally (resistant to) heat, fire and erosion resistant. Due to these properties, asbestos was once widely used in many industrial and construction products. Millions of people have been exposed to asbestos occupationally, environmentally or second hand.

Mesothelioma is caused by inhaling airborne asbestos fibers when ingested into the body. Once the asbestos has entered the body, fibers become lodged in the linings of the lungs, heart or abdomen. Anywhere from 10 to 40 years later, cancerous cells develop in the protective sac linings or mesothelium. Due to the delay between exposure and diagnosis and difficulty identifying symptoms, mesothelioma is often not diagnosed until it has reached later stages. By this time, the prognosis is usually poor, with a median survival time of less than a year.

Currently, there is no known cure for mesothelioma and treatment options are limited to those with advanced disease. Because of this, interventions are not curative but focus on extending survival times and increasing the quality of life. Frontline therapy refers to the first kinds of medical interventions tried and is usually considered the standard clinical practice. Frontline therapies for mesothelioma are surgical resection, chemotherapy, and radiation therapy. An even more common practice is to combine two or more of these methods.

Surgery can include pleurectomy and decortications. Radiation therapy and chemotherapy often follow surgical intervention. Conventional chemotherapy agents used to treat mesothelioma are pemetrexed, cisplatin, carboplatin, doxorubicin, epirubicin, mitomycin, cyclophosphamide, and ifosfamide. Phase II clinical trials have shown success combining cisplatin and pemetrexed in chemotherapy-naive patients, and this combination is now recognized as the preferred first-line treatment for mesothelioma patients.

Surgery, chemotherapy, and radiation treatments are palliative but do not result in extended survival times.

After initial front line treatments have been used, second line therapies can be tried. Clinical trials investigate second line treatments in hopes of finding more efficient ways to fight or even cure mesothelioma. Second line treatments can take the form of new therapeutic drugs, new methods of surgery or radiation or new combinations or continuations of previous frontline approaches. Controlling symptoms or the disease by diet, exercise or alternative healing techniques are considered to be supplementary not front line or secondary methods of treatment.

Not all mesothelioma patients will be eligible for clinical trials researching new therapeutic interventions since they each have their requirements. After completing standard treatments, patients who wish to participate in a clinical trial involving the use of second-line treatments will need to see if they are eligible. Some eligibility requirements are whether the tumors are resectable, whether, or to what extent patients have been pre-treated with pemetrexed or other chemotherapy agents, and what type or stage of the disease the patient currently has.

Second line treatments involving new chemotherapy drugs for mesothelioma are continually being researched. As diagnostic methods improve and mesothelioma is being identified in the earlier stages, second line therapies are increasingly being used for those patients who are still healthy at the time of diagnosis. New drugs, anti-antigenic compounds, molecular antibodies and other alternatives are being tested worldwide. For best results, first and second line treatments should begin right away to achieve the most effective results.

To find out more about current clinical trials investigating both front and second line treatments, consult with your oncologist or mesothelioma specialist to see if you qualify to participate. The National Cancer Institute website is also a useful resource and lists all past and current studies of second-line mesothelioma treatments.

What You Need to Know About Malignant Mesothelioma

Mesothelioma has three principal types. Pleural mesothelioma, which affects the lining of the lungs, is the most common and accounts for approximately 90% of cases. This kind of mesothelioma is usually first recognized by the development of pleural plaques on the lungs. The other two types of mesothelioma are peritoneum, which affects the lining of the abdomen, and pericardium, which affects the lining of the heart. All types of mesothelioma can be either contained to one area or dispersed throughout the body.

Mesothelioma is most common in men. Two-thirds of cases are diagnosed until the later stages of life because it can take decades for symptoms of the disease to develop from the time of initial exposure.

There are three histological types, or microscopic anatomies, of mesothelioma: epithelial, sarcomatous, and biphasic. Epithelial is the most common and refers to tumors that have affected the linings of small cavities in the body. There are different types of epithelium depending on the number of layers and shapes of the cells. Sarcomatous are rarer but more aggressive types of tumors that begin from the connective and muscle tissues.

Exposure to asbestos is the principal cause of mesothelioma. Asbestos is a naturally occurring mineral that was once used in many constructions, industrial, and shipping materials. Most asbestos exposure occurs occupationally, although can occur through contamination of the environment as well.

It's been estimated that more than 8 million workers in the United States alone have been exposed to asbestos. Higher risk occupations include construction, shipyard, and railroad workers as well as mechanics. Secondhand exposure also can occur through household contact with an employee who carries asbestos home on his clothes, hair or skin.

Over 2500 mesothelioma cases are diagnosed per year in the United States, with varying numbers in other countries. The risk is increased for anyone who lives in areas that have higher levels of environmental exposure, such as next to former asbestos mines.

Much research and progress have been made. However, till date no cure for mesothelioma exists. Without treatment, the prognosis from the time of diagnosis is only months, although with treatment can be as long as five years. Longer survival times are associated with epithelial versus sarcomatous or mixed types of mesothelioma.

Diagnosis of mesothelioma is difficult to establish. If you have a known history of exposure to asbestos and are experiencing any adverse health symptoms, consult with your doctor right away. If you have been diagnosed with mesothelioma, find a pathologist or an occupational medicine specialist that you feel comfortable with.

Treating cancer comes with high medical costs. Most patients with mesothelioma have been negligently exposed and are eligible to receive financial compensation. Warnings should have been placed on asbestos-containing products and employers should have protected workers. Therefore, an experienced mesothelioma lawyer can get your monetary help to make up for lost wages and to cover treatments and other associated costs.

Diagnosing mesothelioma in earlier stages makes a difference. If you have any suspicion of exposure to asbestos and are experiencing health problems, contact a specialist for medical advice immediately.

Prevent Mesothelioma: Safety Guidelines Managing Asbestos

Asbestos, known for its thermal and insulating properties, was once widely used in many industrial and construction materials. The carcinogenic nature of asbestos was not discovered until years later. Serious diseases, such as mesothelioma, asbestosis and lung cancers, began to develop in employees and the public decades after exposure. Mesothelioma, the most severe illness, is an incurable cancer that begins when asbestos fibers lodge in the membranes of vital organs. Exposure to asbestos is the primary cause of mesothelioma.

Local, state and federal laws were established in regards to management, repair and removal of asbestos after the dangers of exposure became irrefutable. If the presence of asbestos is set at any construction or home site in the United States, regulations from the following agencies must be followed:

* U.S. Environmental Protection Agency (EPA).

* OSHA: Occupational Safety and Health Administration.

* U.S. Food and Drug Administration (FDA).

* Mine Safety and Health Administration: asbestos safety regulations regarding exposure limits and procedures in line with current OSHA standards.

* CPSC: Consumer Product Safety Commission.

In addition to the federal asbestos abatement laws, local and state agencies also impose their regulations. Such legal efforts were made to prevent harmful and fatal exposure to asbestos. Asbestos removal legislation may vary from state to state and yet most laws require that asbestos abatement is done by licensed professionals who are trained to remove asbestos. Inspection before beginning any demolition, renovation or construction is required before any work can legally begin.

There are three different possibilities if asbestos is discovered during initial inspections: leave it alone, repair it, or remove it.

Asbestos is not considered a risk to health when it is intact and in good condition. It is recommended to leave asbestos materials in good condition alone and undisturbed. However, if the material is damaged or likely to be disturbed, safe repair or removal will be needed.

When a building is undergoing demolition, repair or renovation, asbestos is likely to be disturbed and become airborne. In such situations, local health, environmental and government asbestos regulations will need to be checked. Often, proper and safe repair or removal of asbestos materials will be needed. Recommended repair methods are to seal or cover the original material in such a way that the asbestos is completely contained and concealed. As for removal, most regulating agencies require a certified, trained asbestos abatement company completes an inspection and perform any removal and disposal of materials containing asbestos.

In some situations, plumbing, flooring or roofing contractor may be trained in asbestos removal and meet the requirements to perform abatement activities. Following any and all regulations regarding the proper and safe removal and disposal of asbestos will prevent anyone from facing serious criminal charges or fines. More importantly, any chance of exposure to asbestos and developing mesothelioma will be avoided, and the health and safety of all will be protected.

Receiving a diagnosis of malignant mesothelioma is a heartbreaking and painful experience for the patient as well as for family and loved ones. It can feel shocking as if your whole world has been turned upside down. Many feel anger, loss of control, and overwhelm when first told they have a diagnosis of terminal mesothelioma cancer.

Mesothelioma is cancer primarily caused by exposure to asbestos. Asbestos is a fibrous mineral that was well known for being durable, fire resistant, and a superb, multi-purposed insulator. Because of these properties, and its affordability and availability, asbestos was used in many commercial, manufacturing, and industrial products, causing many people to be exposed occupationally as well as environmentally.

Asbestos, when inhaled or ingested, causes serious and fatal illnesses. Mesothelioma is one type of incurable cancer caused by inhaling asbestos, which then becomes lodged in the lining of the lungs, chest or abdomen. Mesothelioma is often not diagnosed until decades later because of a long latency period between the time of first exposure and development of symptoms.

Despite the improvement in diagnostic methods and increased knowledge about mesothelioma, symptoms are difficult to diagnose and often the terminal cancer is not diagnosed until it has reached advanced stages. Most patients diagnosed with mesothelioma have a short life expectancy, although research into new drugs and treatments holds a promise of lengthening survival times and quality of life.

For the patient as well as loved ones, it can be tough to face and cope with a terminal diagnosis of malignant mesothelioma. Common feelings associated with the initial diagnosis are denial, anger, shock and grief. While some will resist and deny the reality of having a terminal illness, others will reach a stage of acceptance. Exploring end of life concerns and wishes often forces patients and loved ones to face a variety of emotions and concerns.

Some coping tips to help and to empower during this time are:

1. Inform yourself: learn as much as possible about mesothelioma, the causes, what type and which stage you have been diagnosed with. Also, find out as much as possible about standard, frontline treatments as well as alternative therapies and latest drug research. If you are overwhelmed, resigned, or too upset, ask for a loved one to help you research your illness. Explore the possibility of participating in a clinical trial, which accepts eligible patients and tries new treatment methods with the aim of extending survival time and improving the quality of life. Ask your mesothelioma specialist about any clinical trials in the area and about your eligibility to join.

2. Find support: build a network of support, including not only friends and family but also doctors, specialists, palliative and hospice care, e.t.c. Make sure to include someone you can talk to about your concerns and fears about your cancer and death and dying. People who can offer emotional, physical, and spiritual support will be needed. Surround yourself with those that can show compassion and be helpful, and avoid those that can be emotionally draining or cause upset or anxiety. Do not be afraid to ask for exactly what you need and communicate that to those caring for you. Also, learn about hospice and palliative care, both

of which will give you more choice about how and where you will spend your remaining time and significantly increase your quality of life on all levels.

3. Learn about your sources of medical benefits and legal compensation: Know your medical and health benefits and what is covered by your insurance. Also, anyone diagnosed with mesothelioma should consult with an experienced asbestos attorney to receive additional financial compensation to help with the loss of wages and treatment costs. Manufacturers knew of the dangers of asbestos since at least the early 1960's if not before and yet failed to warn or protect workers and the public from exposure and illness. A mesothelioma attorney who specializes in filing asbestos lawsuits will be able to help you identify the source of your exposure and be successful in maximizing your financial recovery.

4. Explore local and on-line support groups: Treatment centers usually have support groups that hold regular meetings. If a local group is not available, national and on-line support is also available and can provide many resources. Often joining a support group and hearing others share their experiences helps someone newly diagnosed learn more information and gain confidence in sharing their concerns and wishes.

5. Take care of yourself, your family, and your relationships: In such a difficult time, it will be very beneficial to take the time to spend with your loved ones. For some, it is a time to have

meaningful conversations and to heal any past grievances, regrets or upsets. Remembering good times, laughter, and non-cancer conversations can help relieve stress and ease pain, fear, and anxiety.

Most patients and their families will realize that even with new treatments and drug therapies, mesothelioma cannot be cured, although life can be extended and quality of life can be improved. Taking steps like those listed above can help mesothelioma patients and their loved ones realize that despite not being able to change the diagnosis, they do have some choice about how to move forward in treating the illness that can make a difference.

Conclusion

Today, there are many types of cancers that are very well known, like liver, pancreatic, or breast cancer that cannot be prevented. But, did you know that there is only one form of cancer that is entirely 100% preventable, it is called mesothelioma? Mesothelioma symptoms are very similar to all kinds of common ailments, which is one of the reasons that it is rarely detected soon enough by the doctors so that the patient's life can be saved.

The reason that mesothelioma cancer could be totally eradicated off the face of the earth, if only our governments were dedicated enough, is that it is caused by coming in contact with a single substance. The material that causes this form of cancer is called asbestos.

Mankind has known about and used asbestos for 1,000's of years. In the United States, mining for it began in the mid-1800s. By the 20th century, it was being used to manufacture all kinds of products for the general public. Although it was suspected of harming humans for quite some time, it was not until much later that it was scientifically proven to cause mesothelioma cancer.

The most common mesothelioma cancer symptoms are the following, shortness of breath, pain in the chest area, and a cough that is very persistent which will not go away. Some of the other symptoms that this disease displays are high fever, sweating at night while you are sleeping, and the loss of lots of weight.

If you read all of the above mesothelioma cancer symptoms very carefully, you would realize that they are the same exact warning signs, that many other less serious illnesses exhibits. This is one of the reasons that most family doctors have a tough time of correctly diagnosing it on your first visit to their office.

If you believe that you somehow can in contact with asbestos, and showing any signs of the symptoms mentioned above, you really should schedule an appointment with your doctor as soon as possible. When you go to see them, you want to make sure to let them know that you think you were around asbestos.

The next thing you want to let them know are the mesothelioma cancer symptoms that you are experiencing. Finally, you want to make sure that you ask them to test for the disease immediately.

There are very few people that have ever survived having mesothelioma cancer. The few fortunate ones that do were the ones where it was caught very early in its developmental process, and the doctors were able to treat it successfully. By the time it develops into stage III cancer, there is little or nothing that the physicians can do for you other than supply, you very strong pain medication, which will make your last few days less stressful.

Please make sure that if you were around asbestos and you are showing any of the above mesothelioma cancer symptoms, that you go to your doctor, and get yourself thoroughly checked out and tested.

Thank you for downloading my book it is my firm believe that you will apply the acquired knowledge productively.

Check Out Other Books

Go here to check out other books that might interest you:

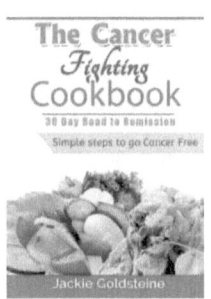

The Cancer Fighting Cookbook: 30 Day Road to Remission

http://amzn.to/28PcS66

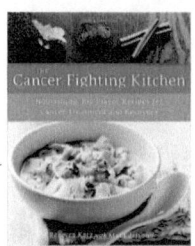

The Cancer-Fighting Kitchen: Nourishing, Big-Flavor Recipes for Cancer Treatment and Recovery

http://amzn.to/28Rn67i

www.ingramcontent.com/pod-product-compliance
Lightning Source LLC
Chambersburg PA
CBHW021446170526
45164CB00001B/419